A IS FOR ASSISTANT

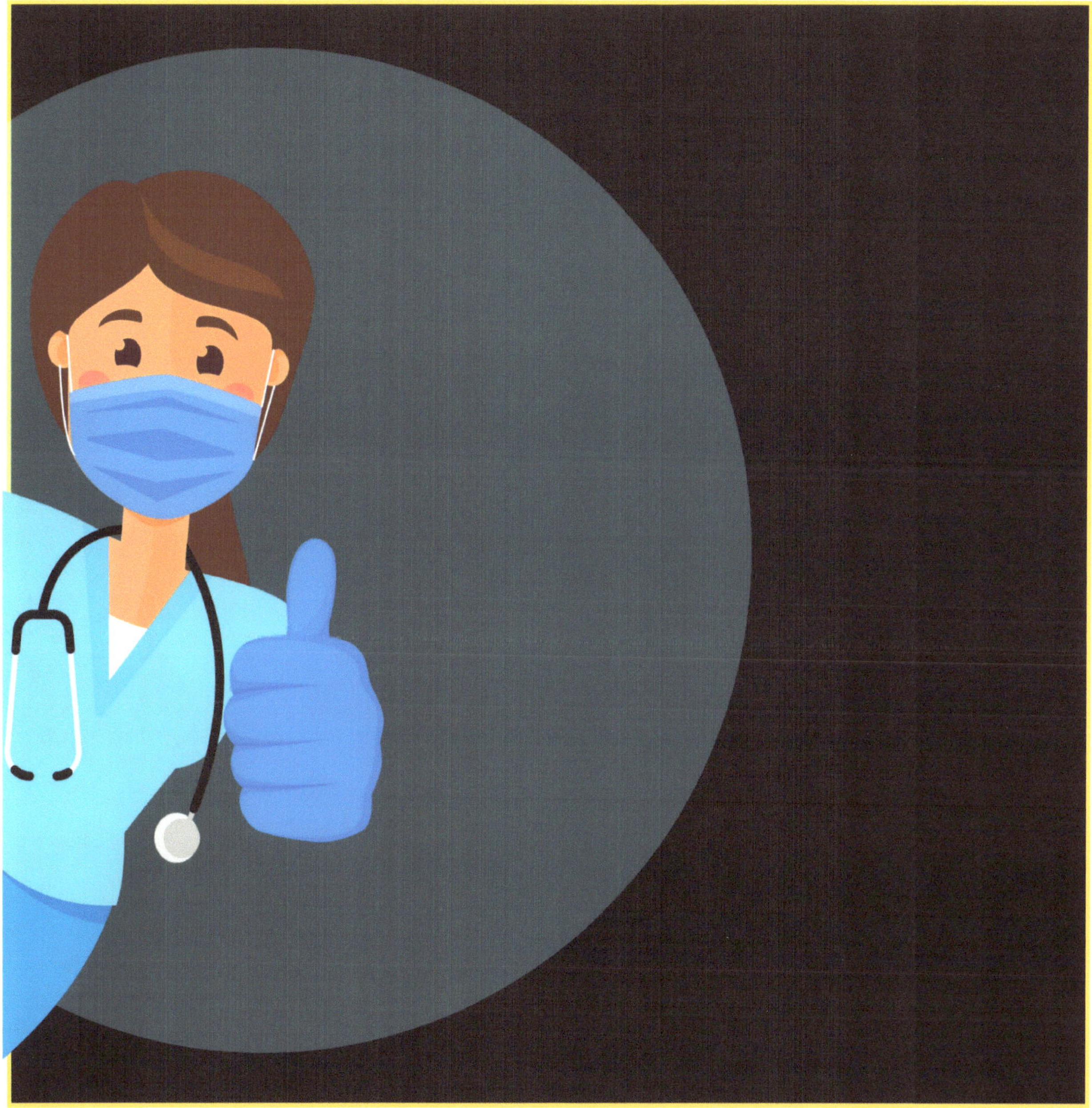

B IS FOR BRIDGE

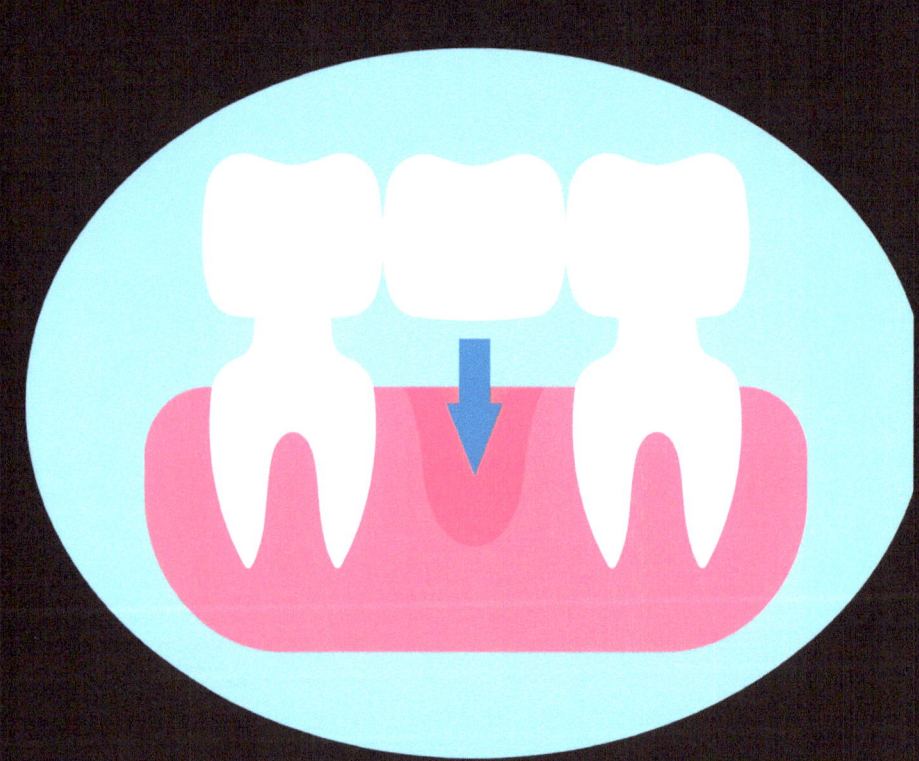

Fills a gap in between teeth

C IS FOR CAVITY

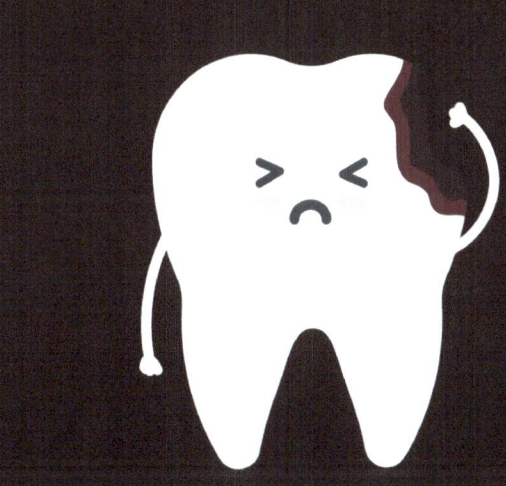

& CROWN

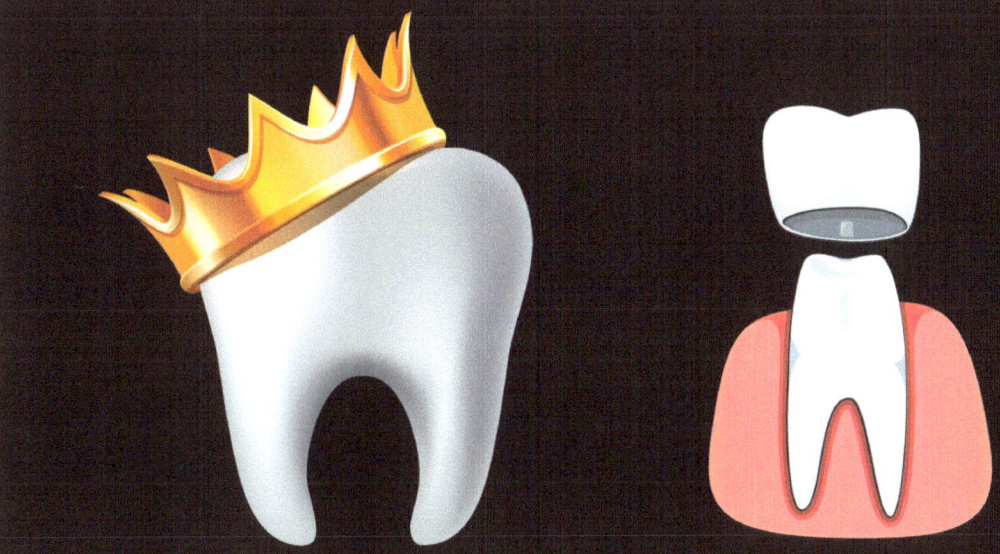

D IS FOR DENTIST

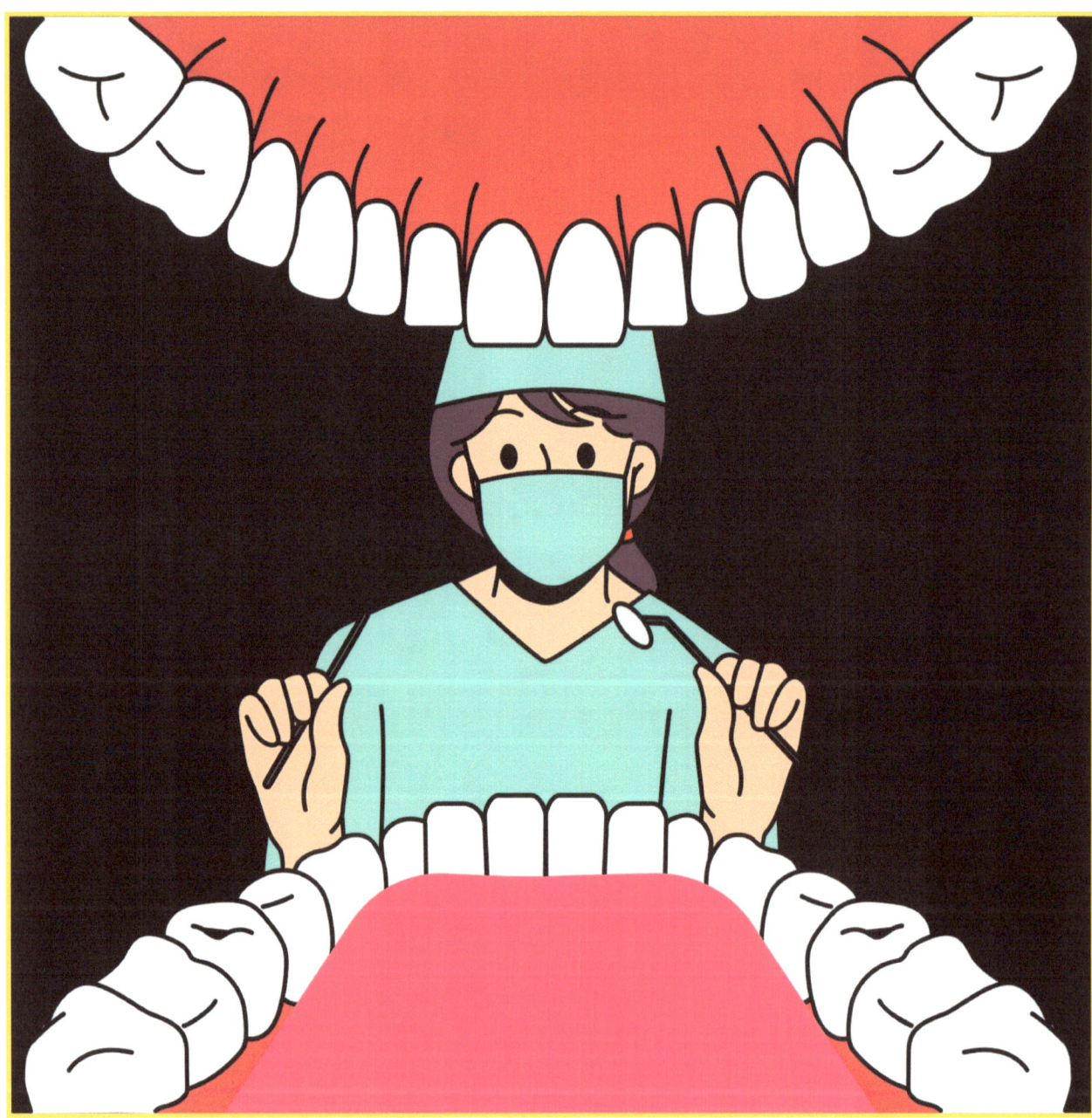

E IS FOR ENAMEL

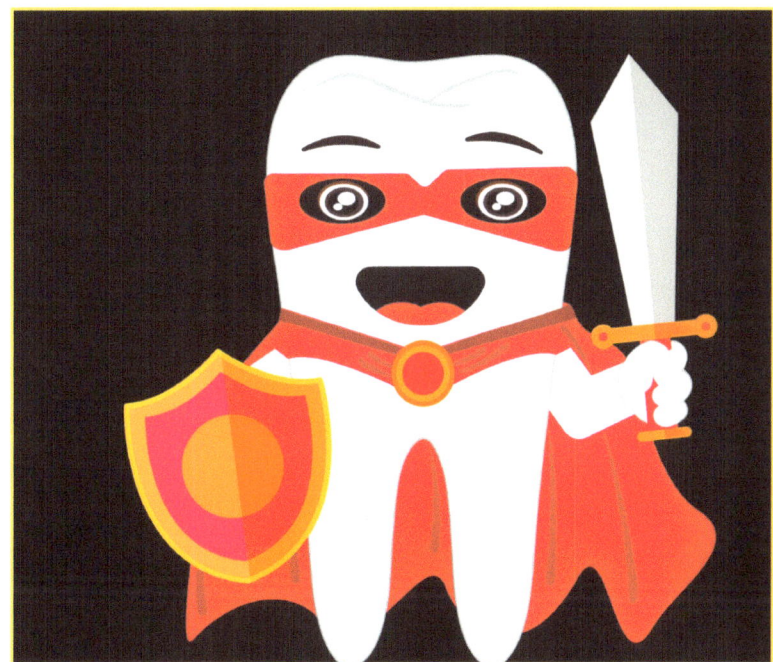

&

EXTRACTION

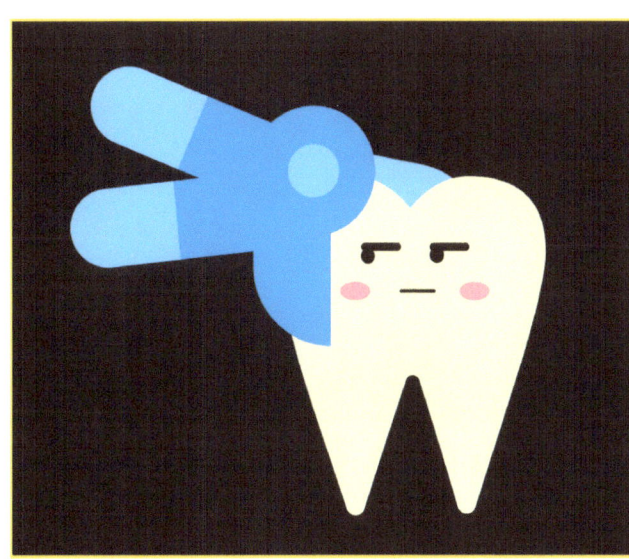

F IS FOR FLOSS

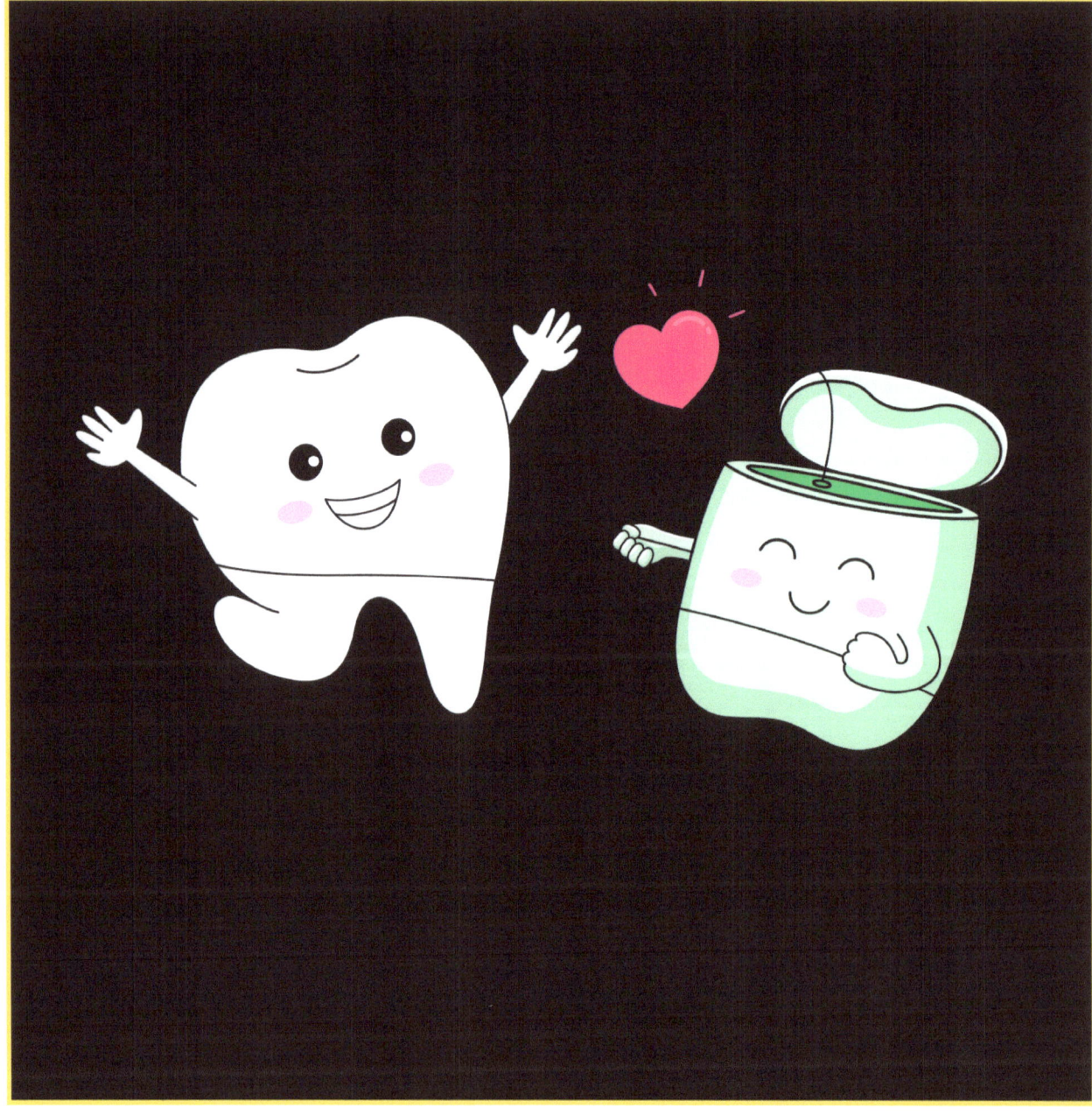

G IS FOR GINGIVA

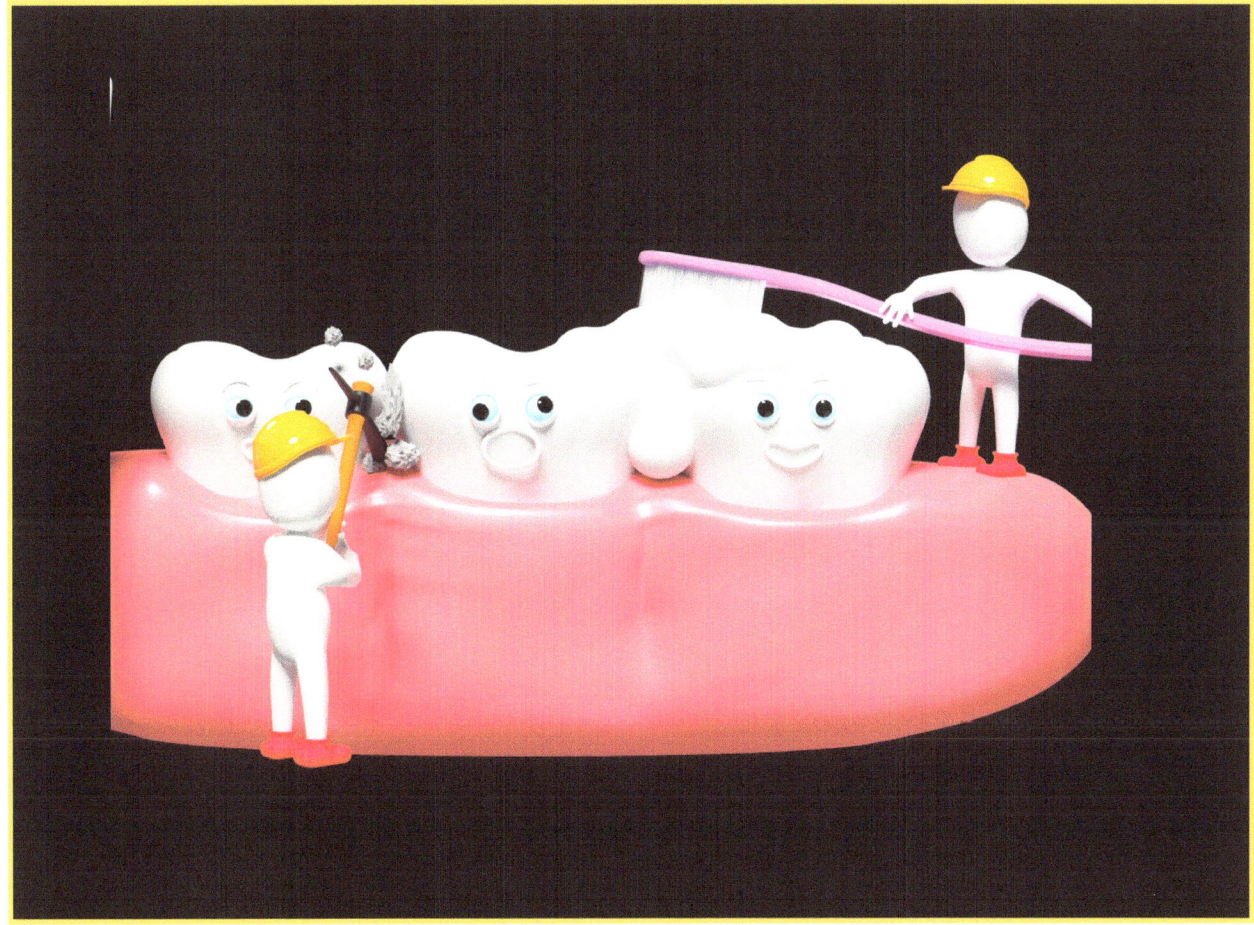

A.K.A. GUMS

H IS FOR HYGIENIST

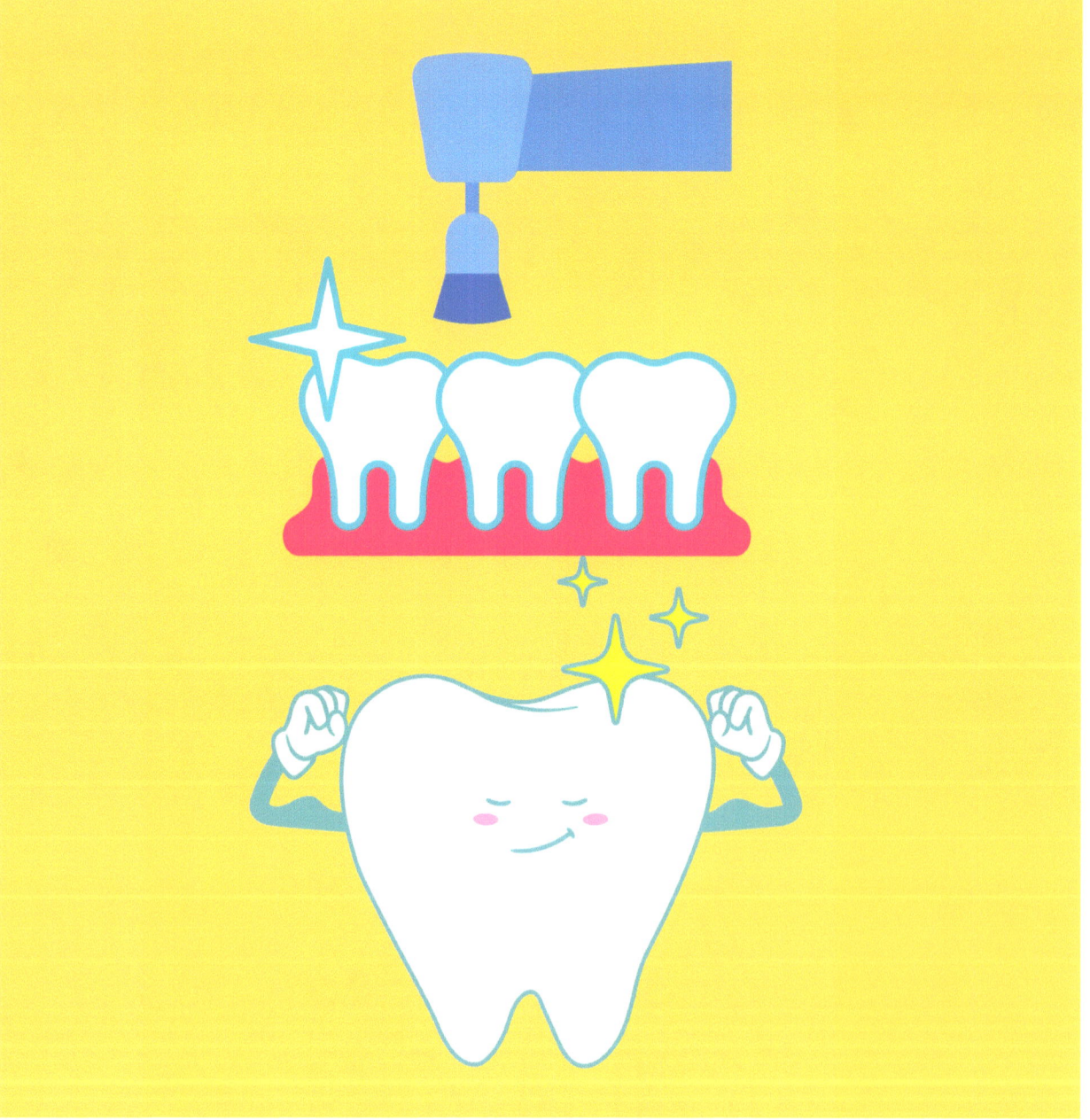

I IS FOR IMPLANTS

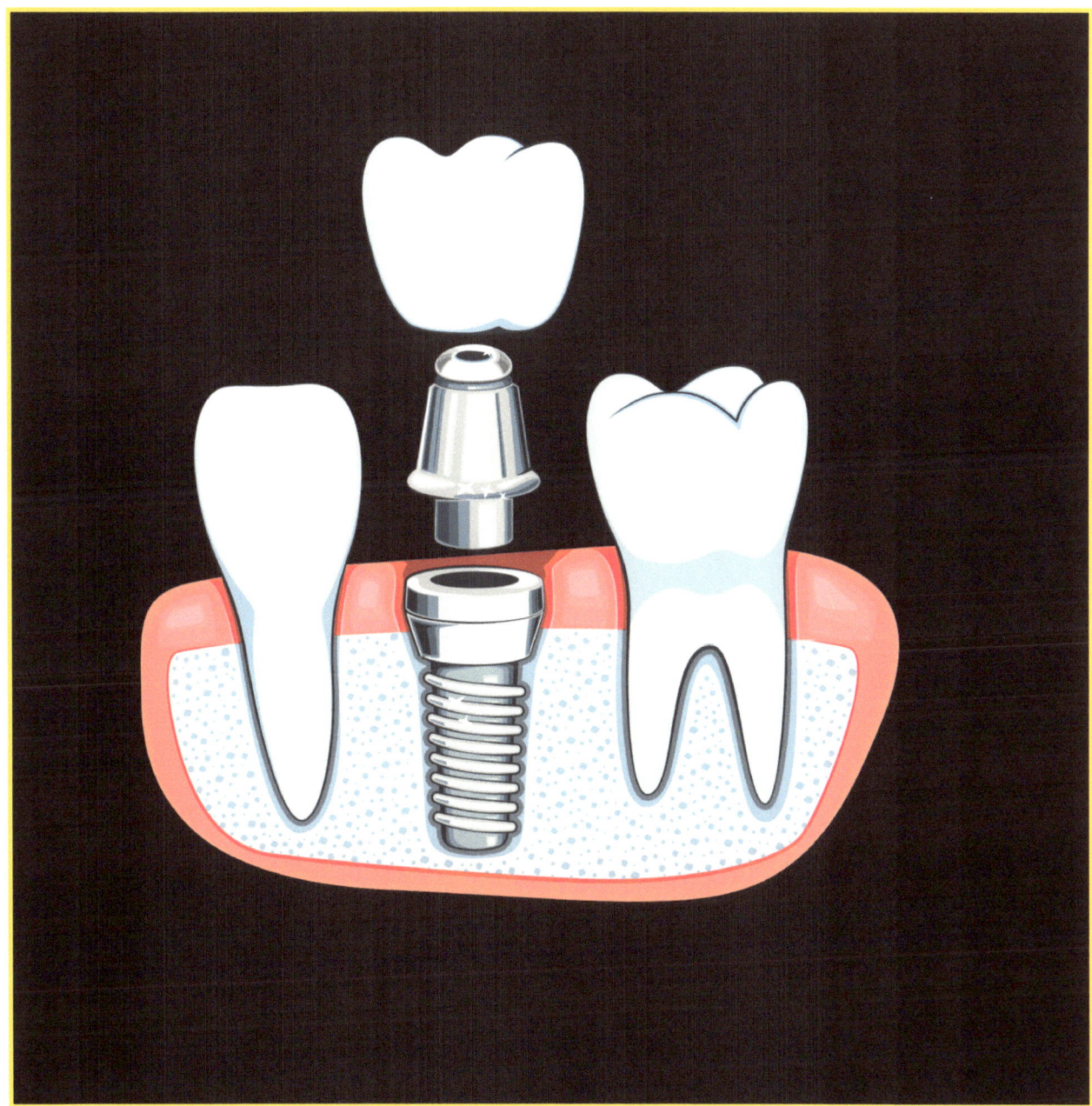

J IS FOR JAW

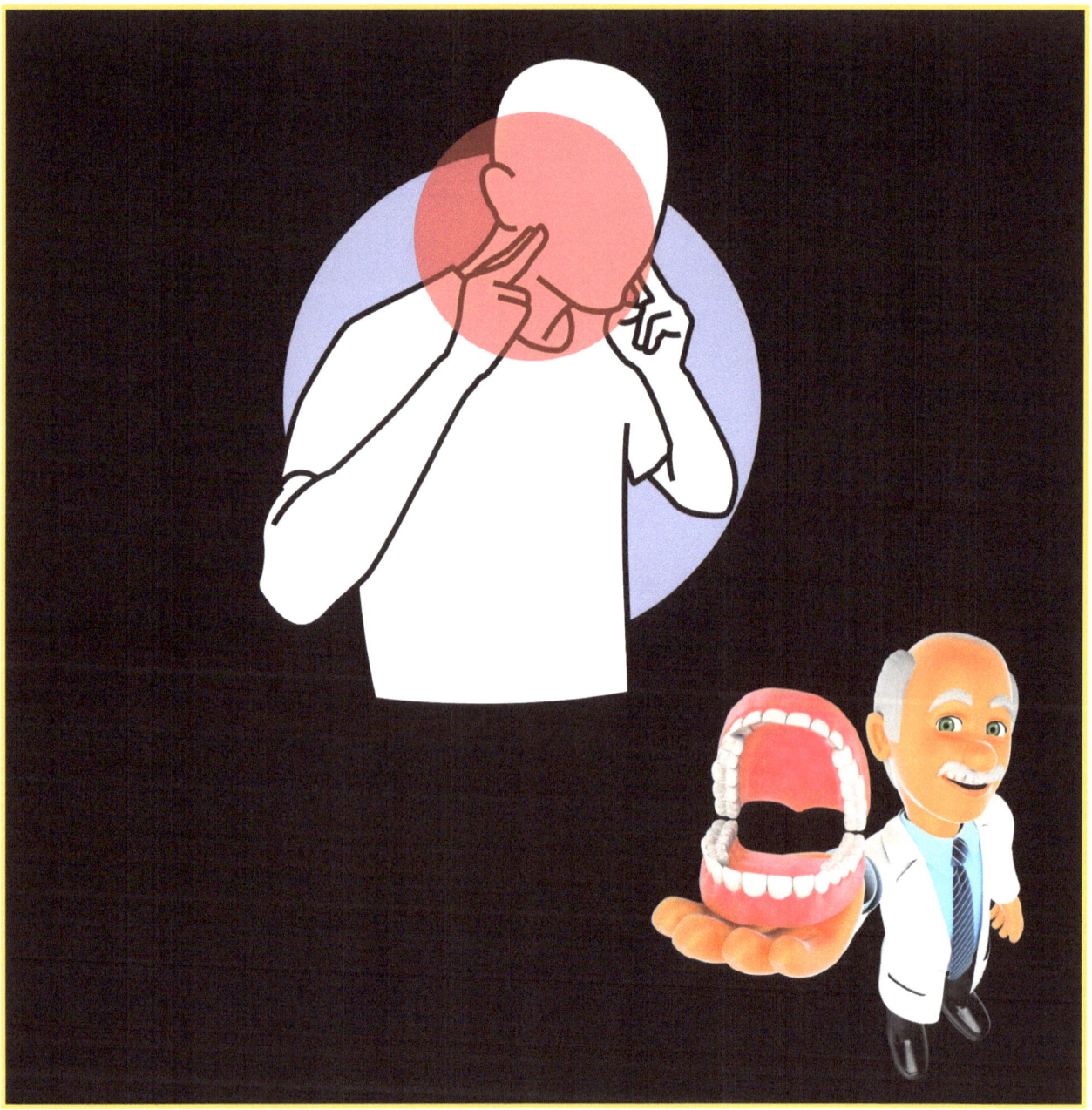

K IS FOR KIDS

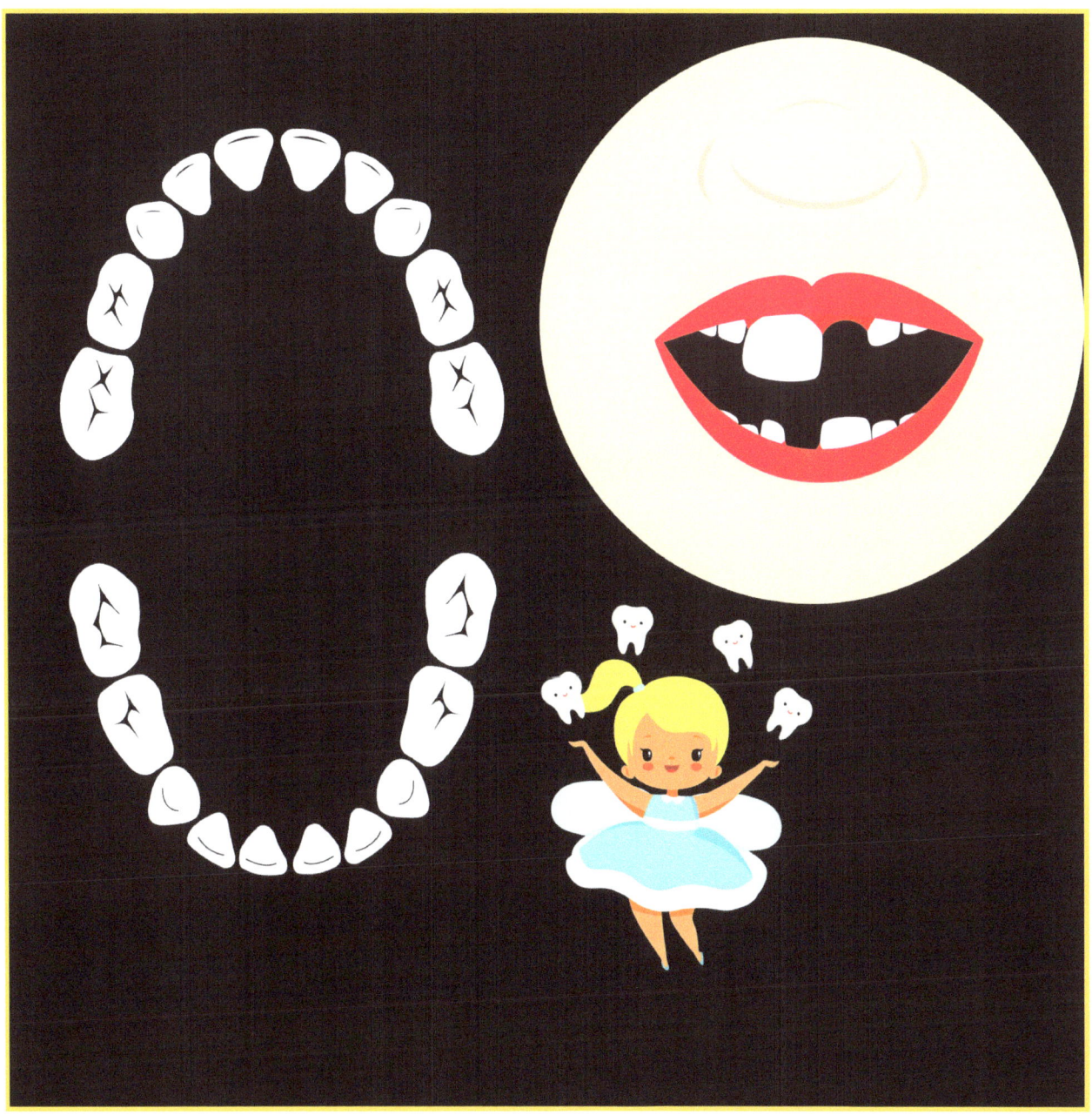

L IS FOR LABORATORY

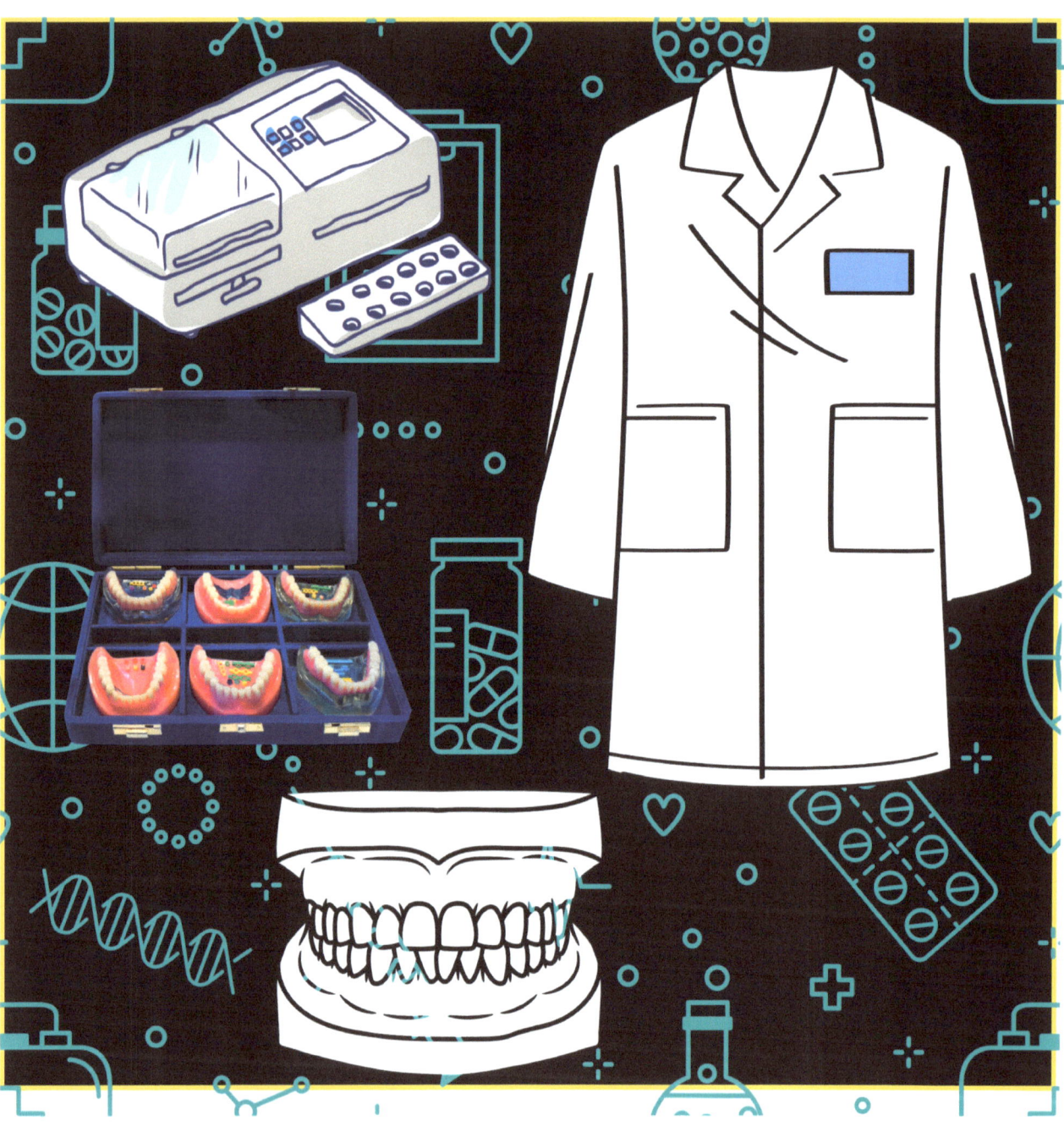

M IS FOR MIRROR

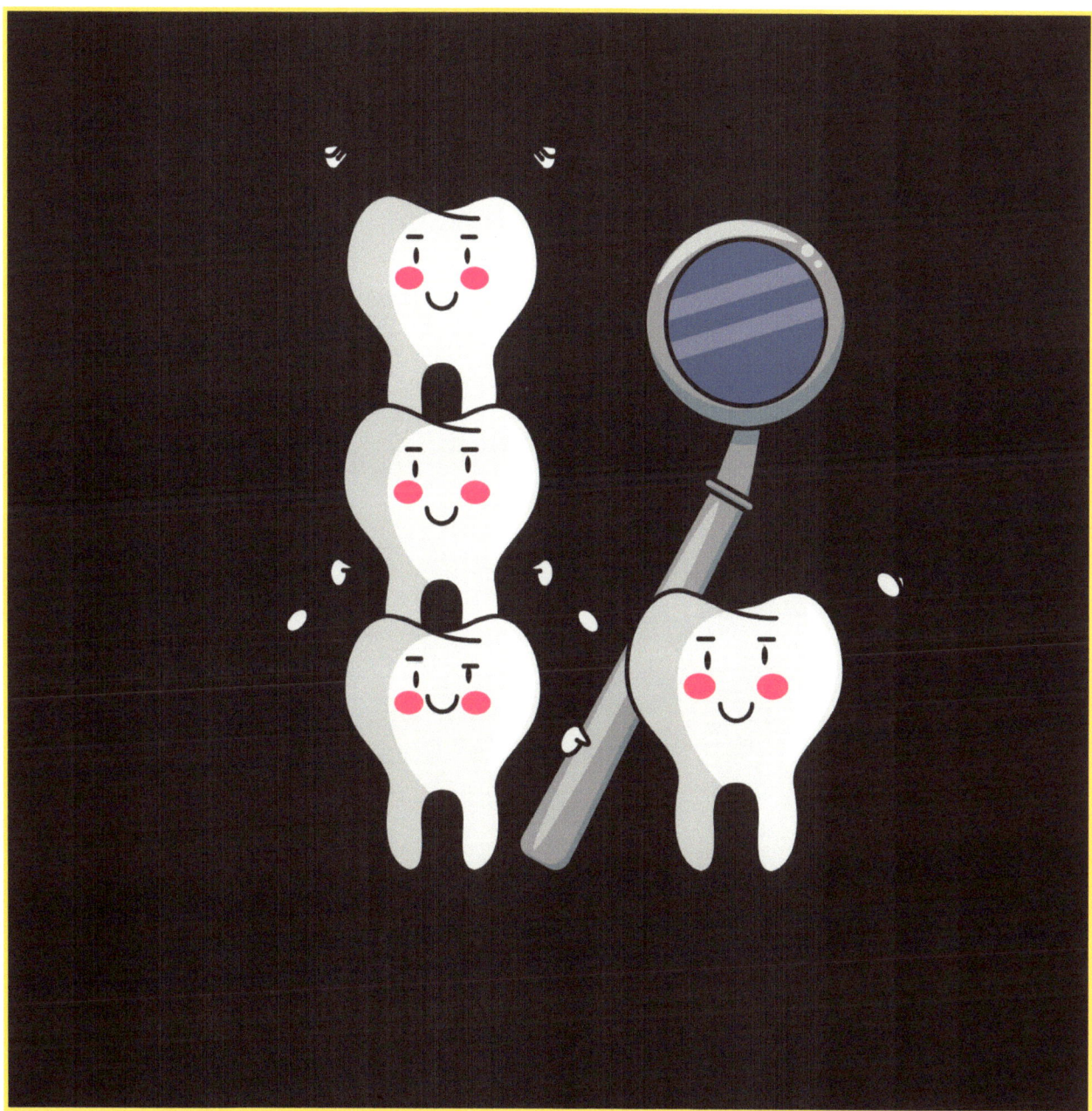

N IS FOR NIGHTGUARD

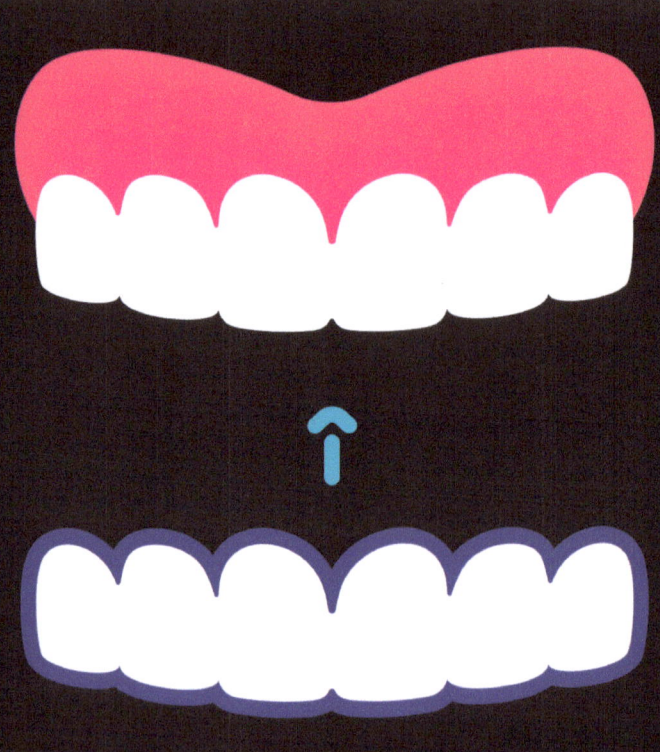

Helps with Bruxism (Grinding)

O IS FOR ORTHODONTICS

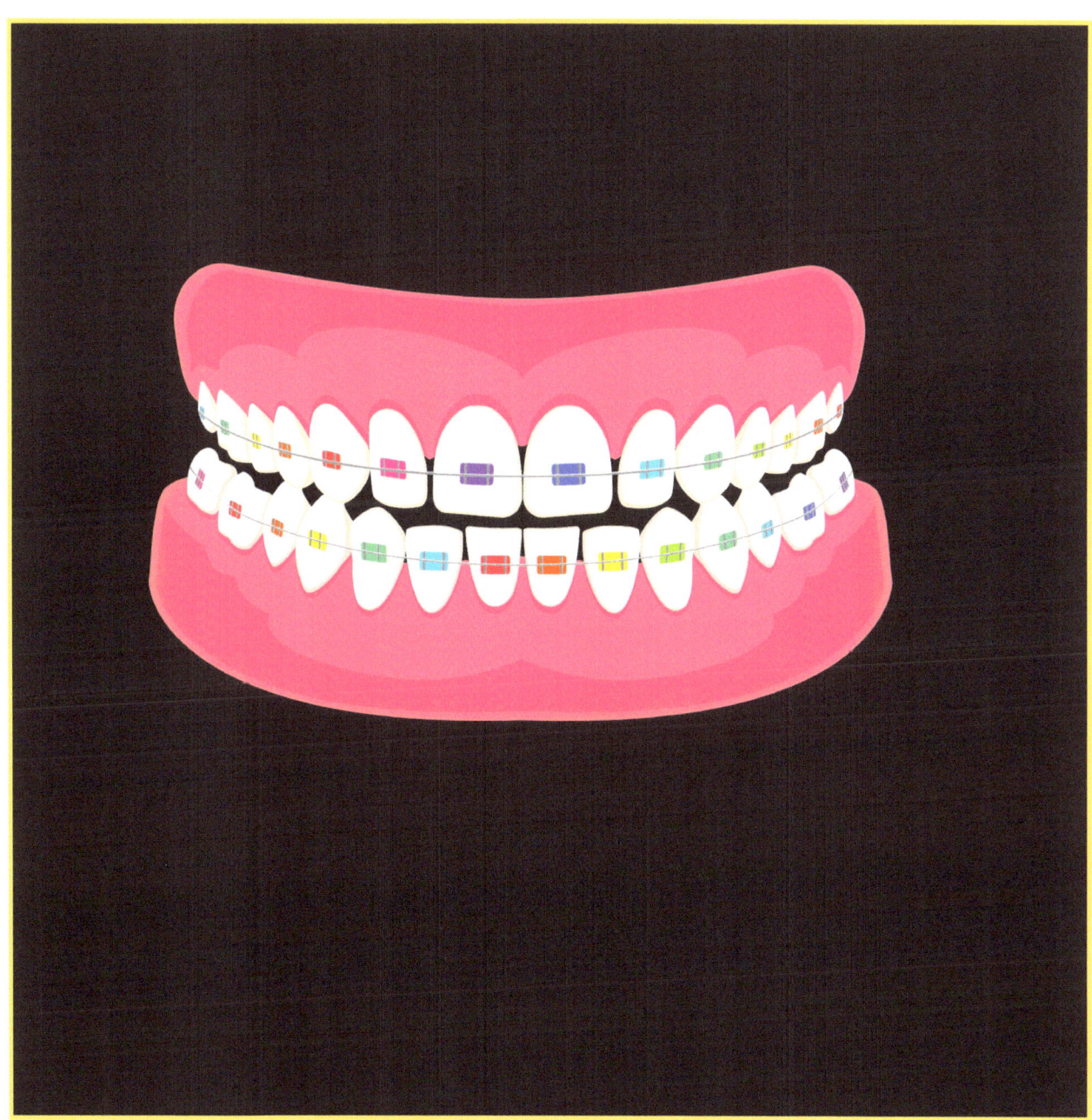

P IS FOR PANORAMIC

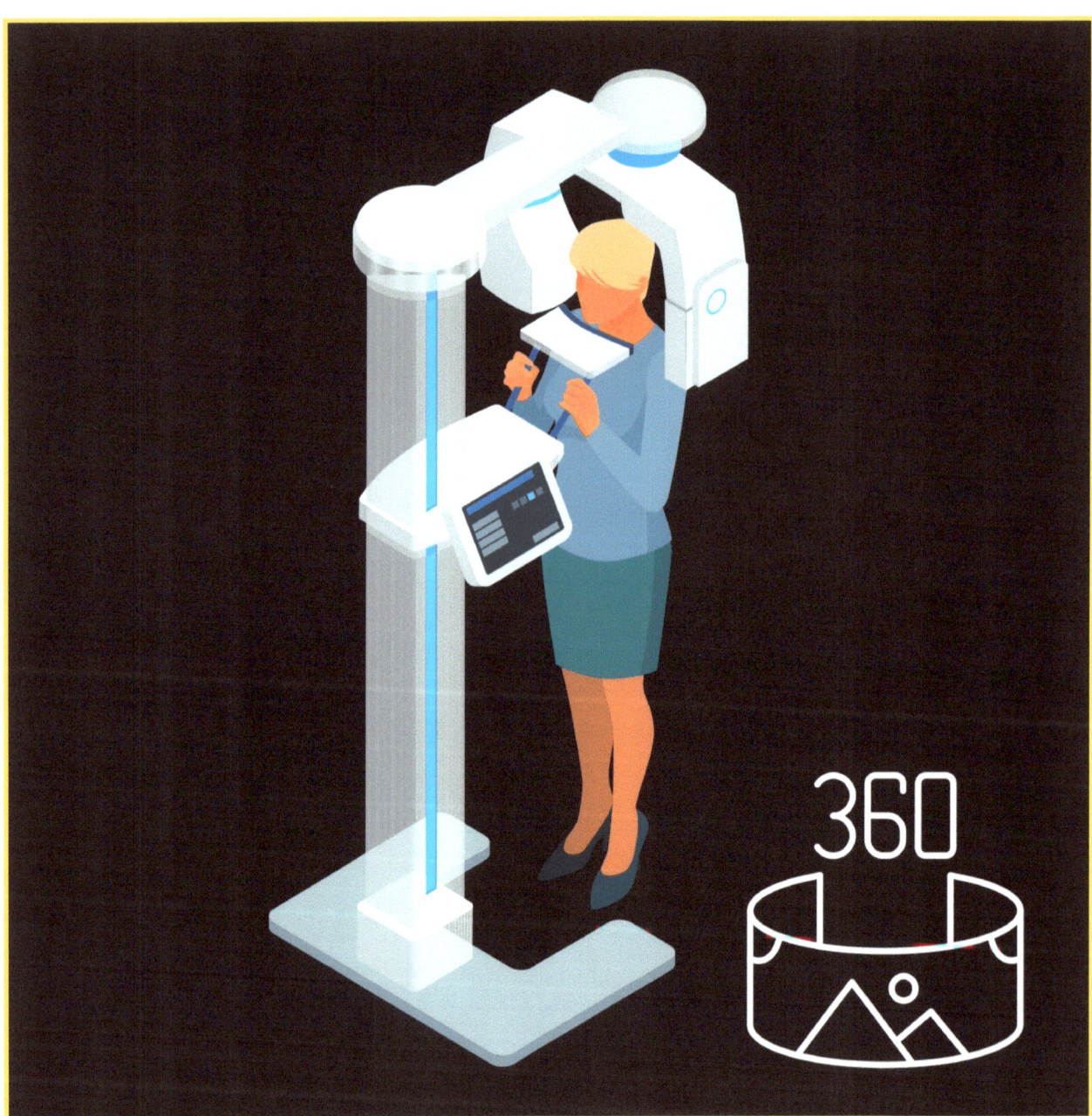

Q IS FOR QUADRANT

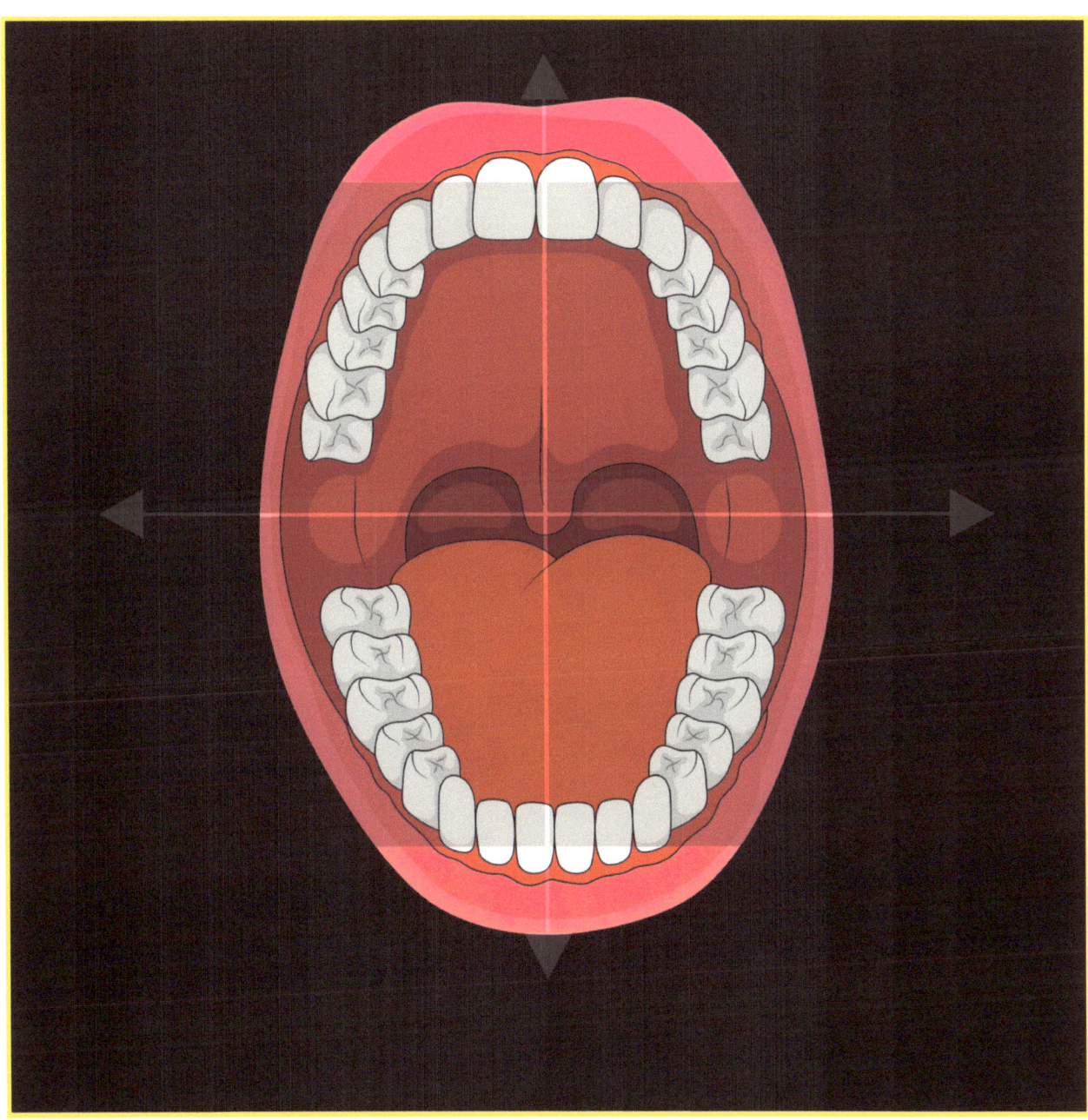

R IS FOR RESTORATION

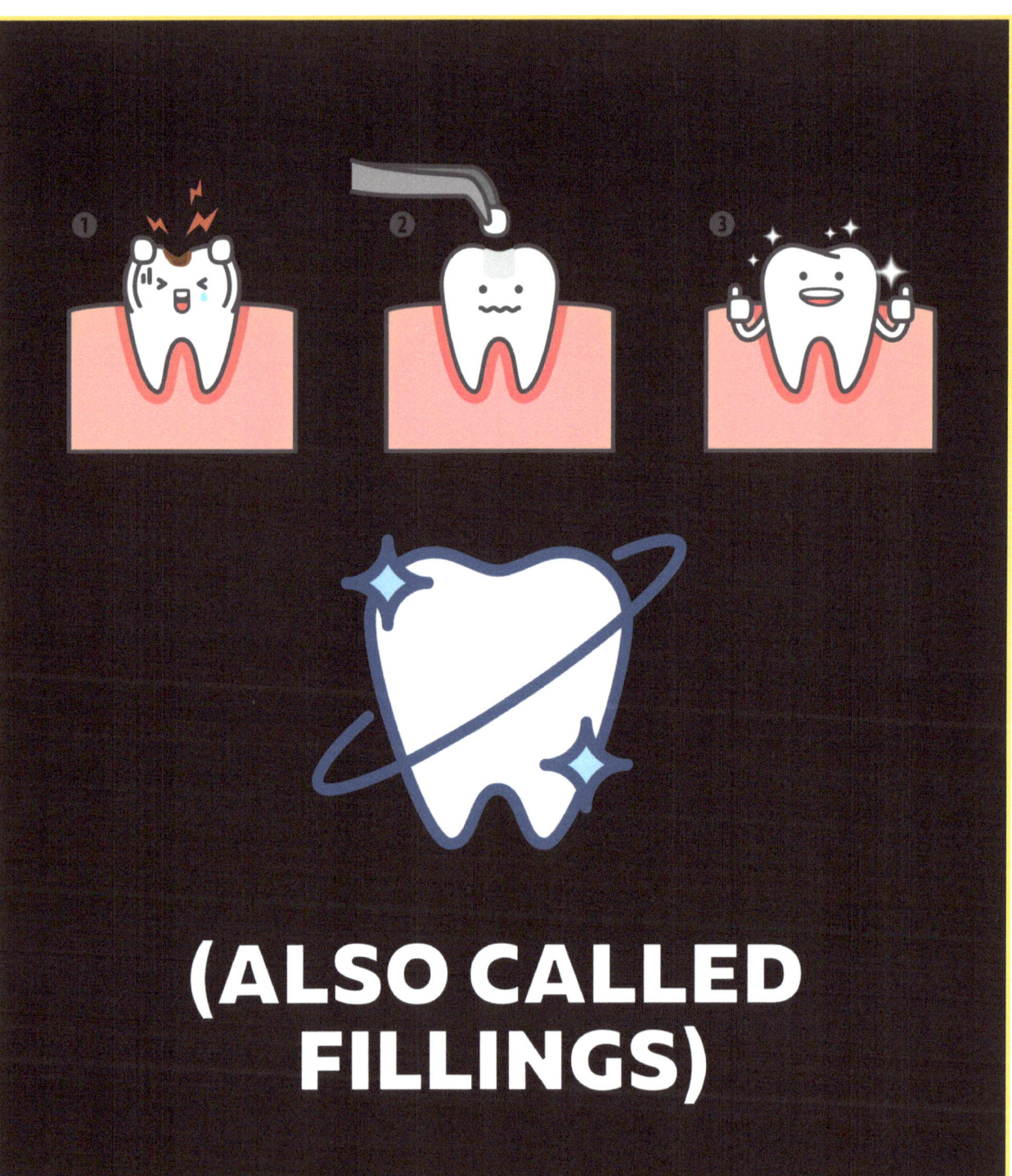

(ALSO CALLED FILLINGS)

R IS ALSO FOR ROOT CANAL

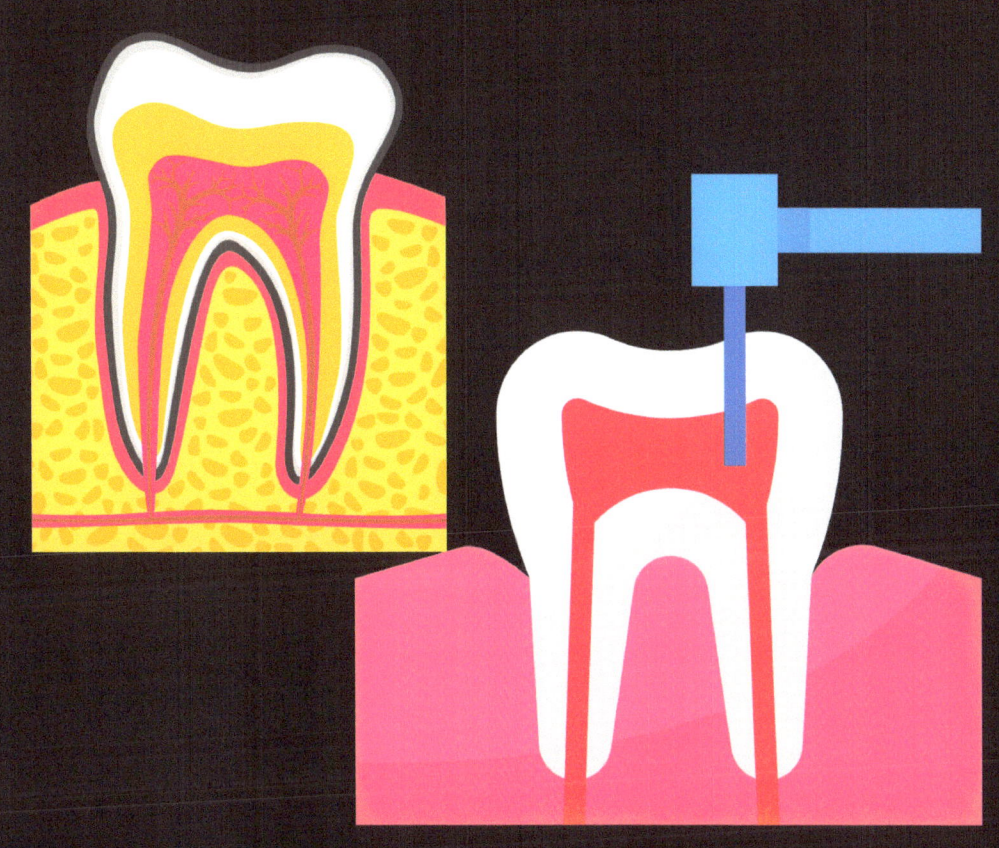

WHICH IS ALSO CALLED ENDODONTICS

S IS FOR SCALING

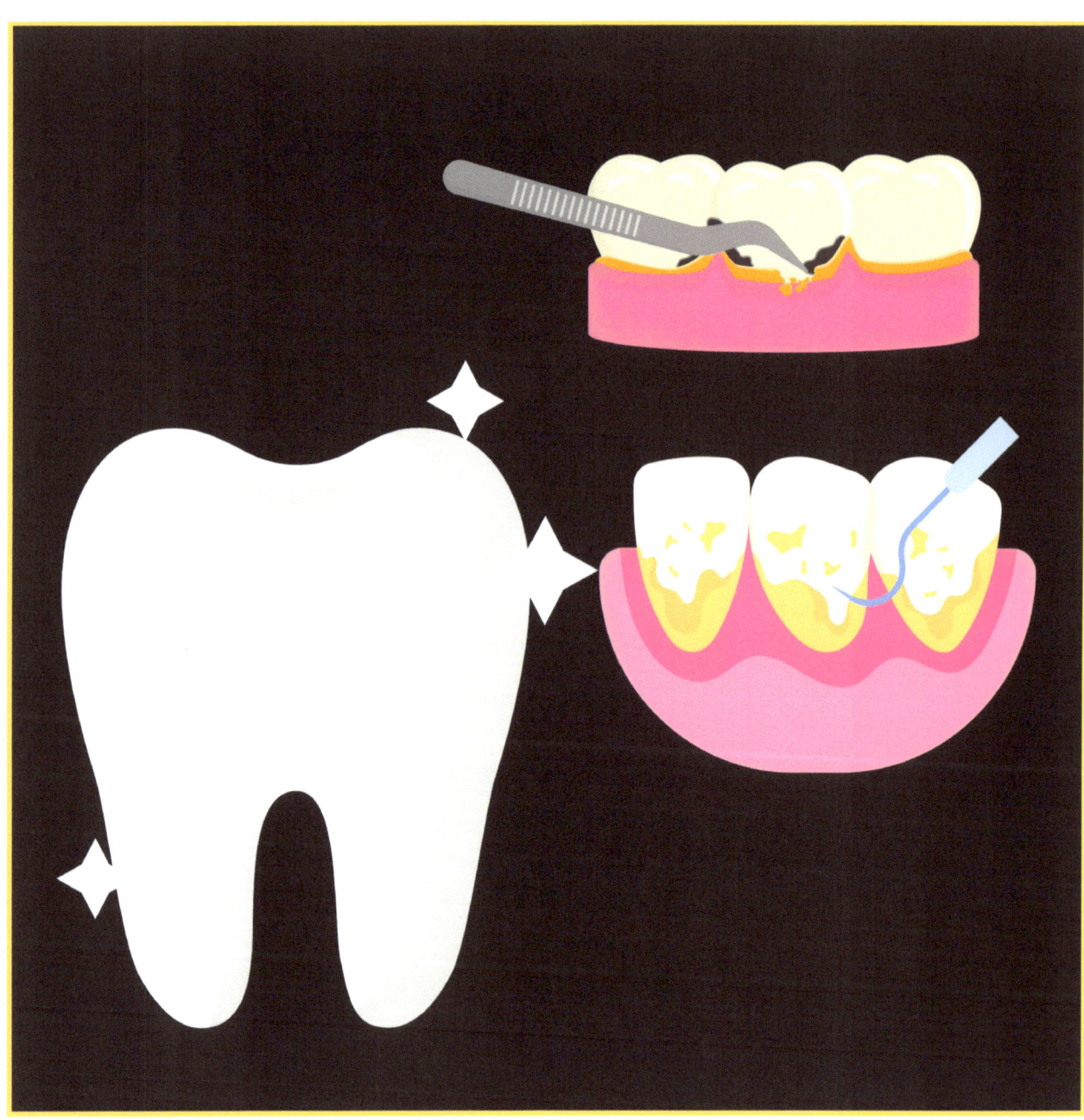

T IS FOR TEETH

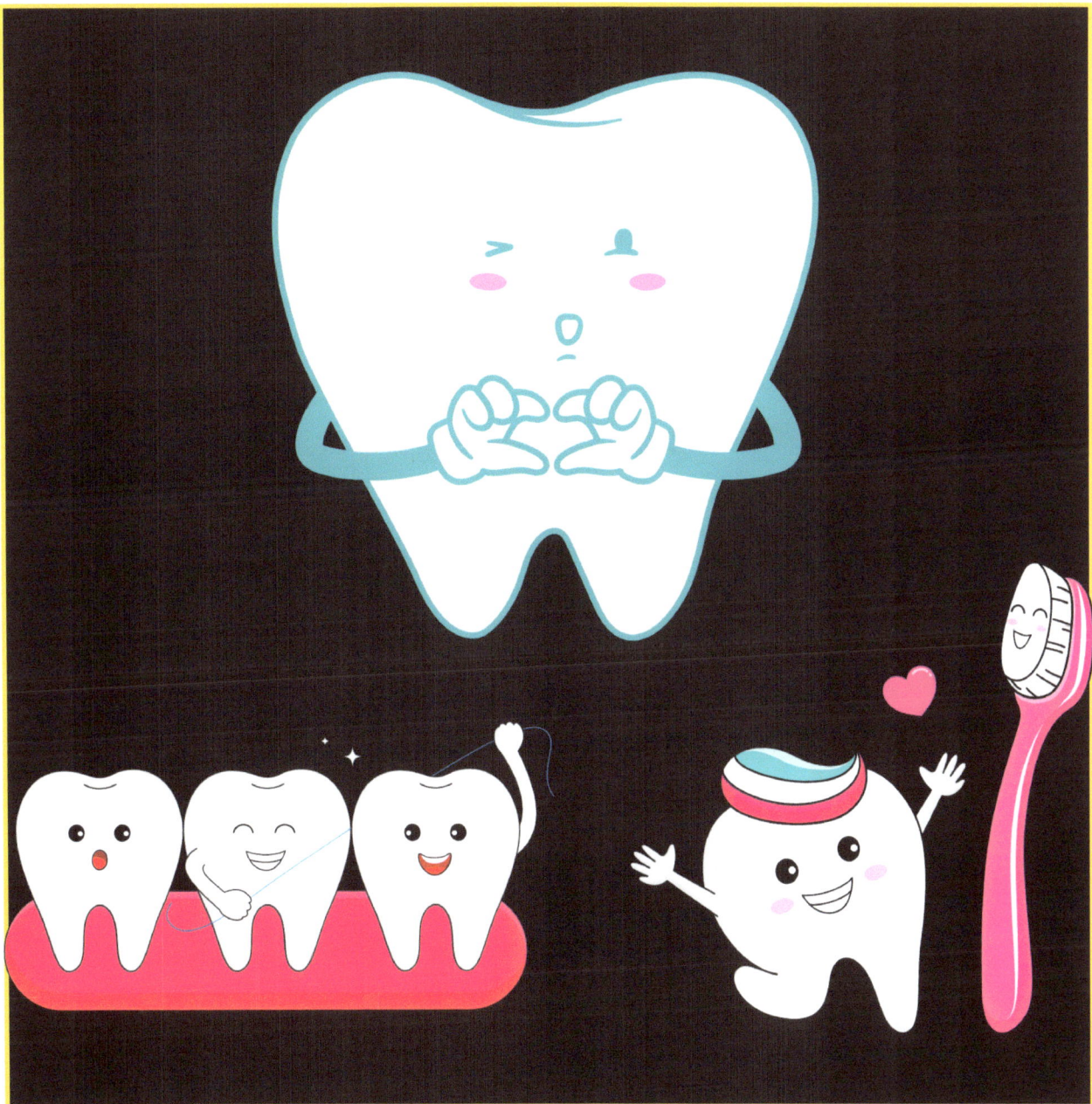

U IS FOR ULTRASONIC

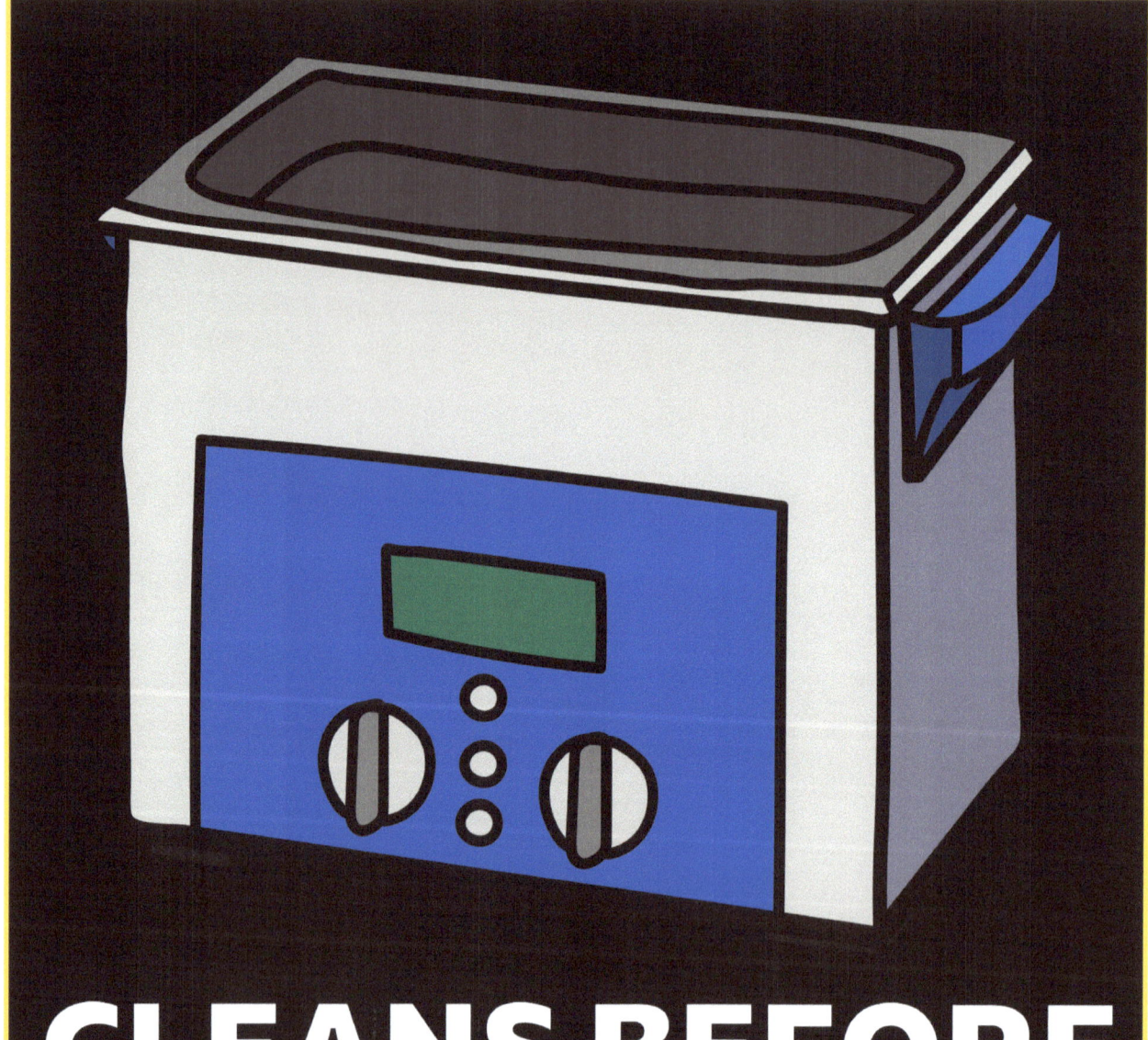

CLEANS BEFORE STERLIZATION

V IS FOR VENEER

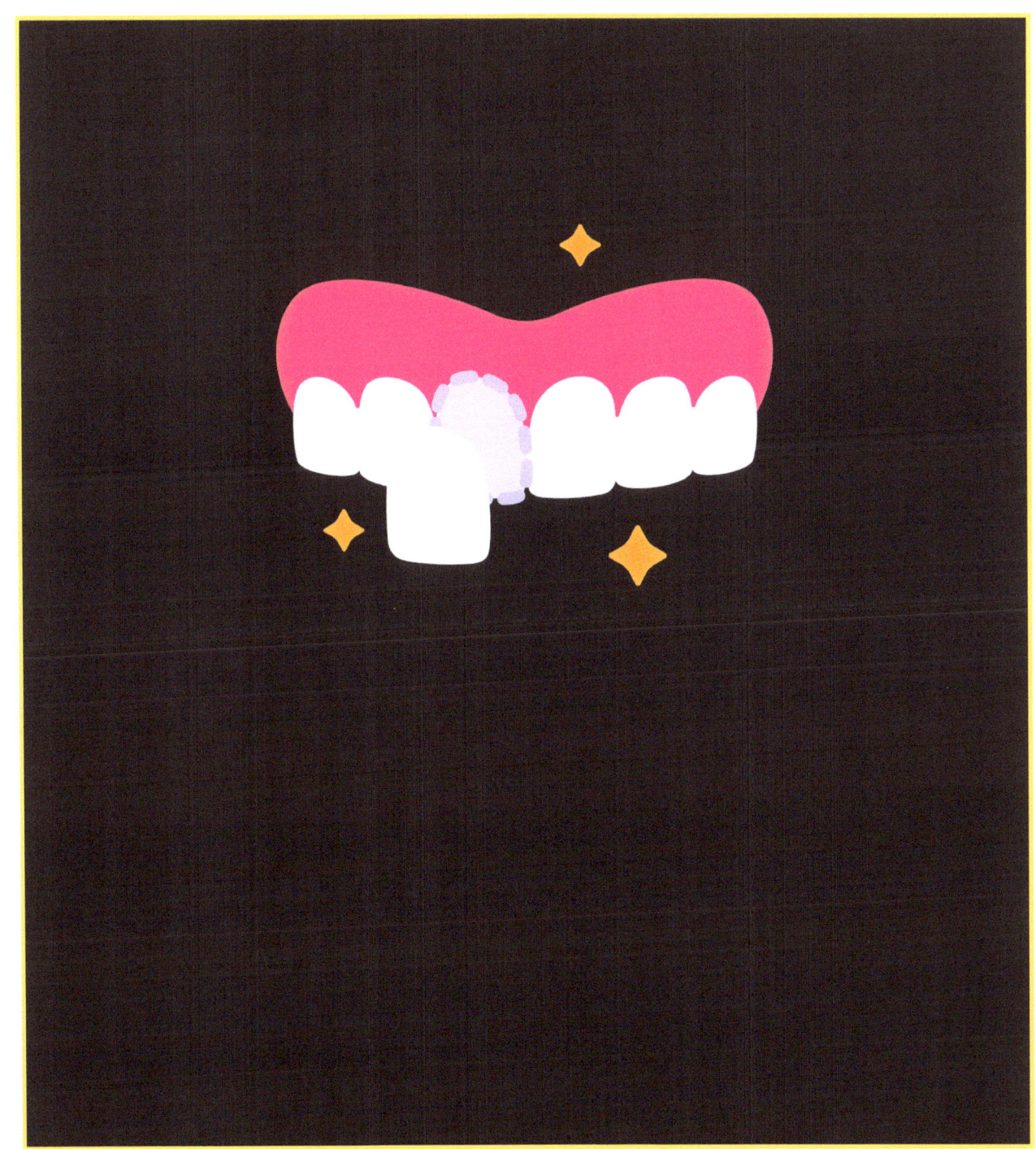

W IS FOR WHITENING

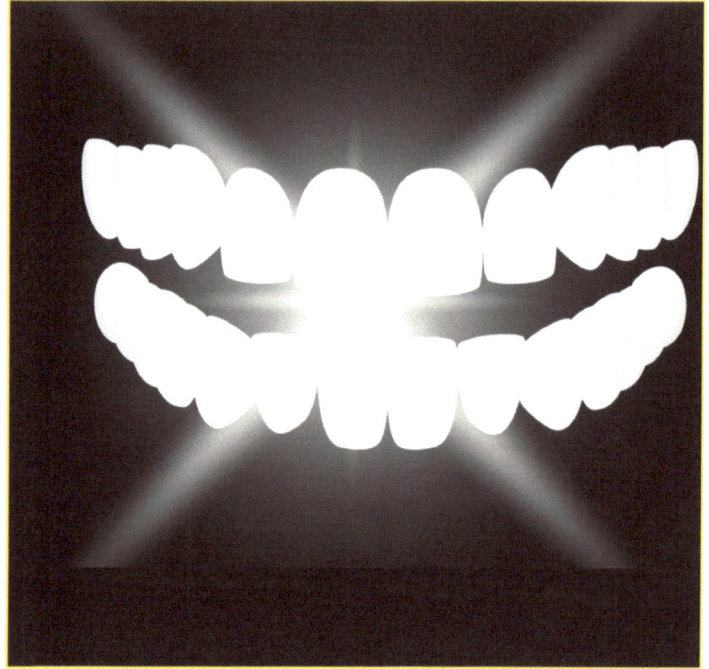

& WISDOM TEETH

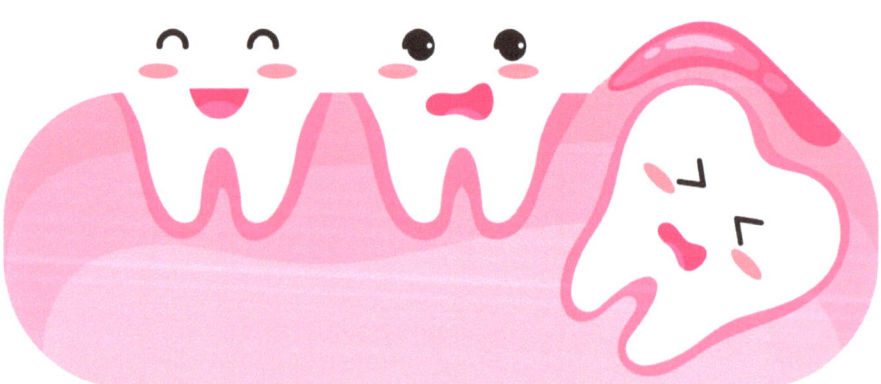

X IS FOR X-RAY

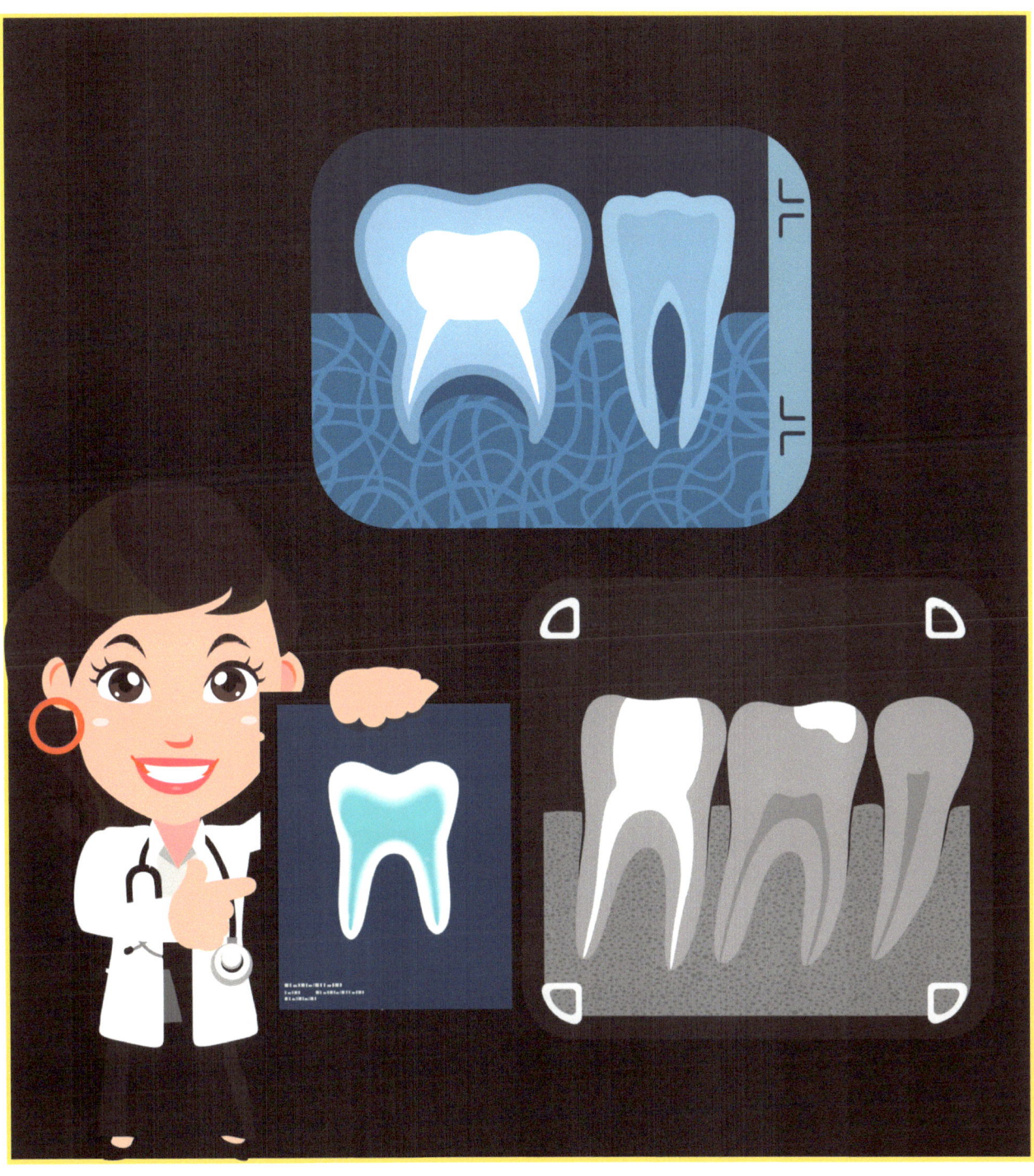

Y IS FOR YOUR ORAL HEALTH

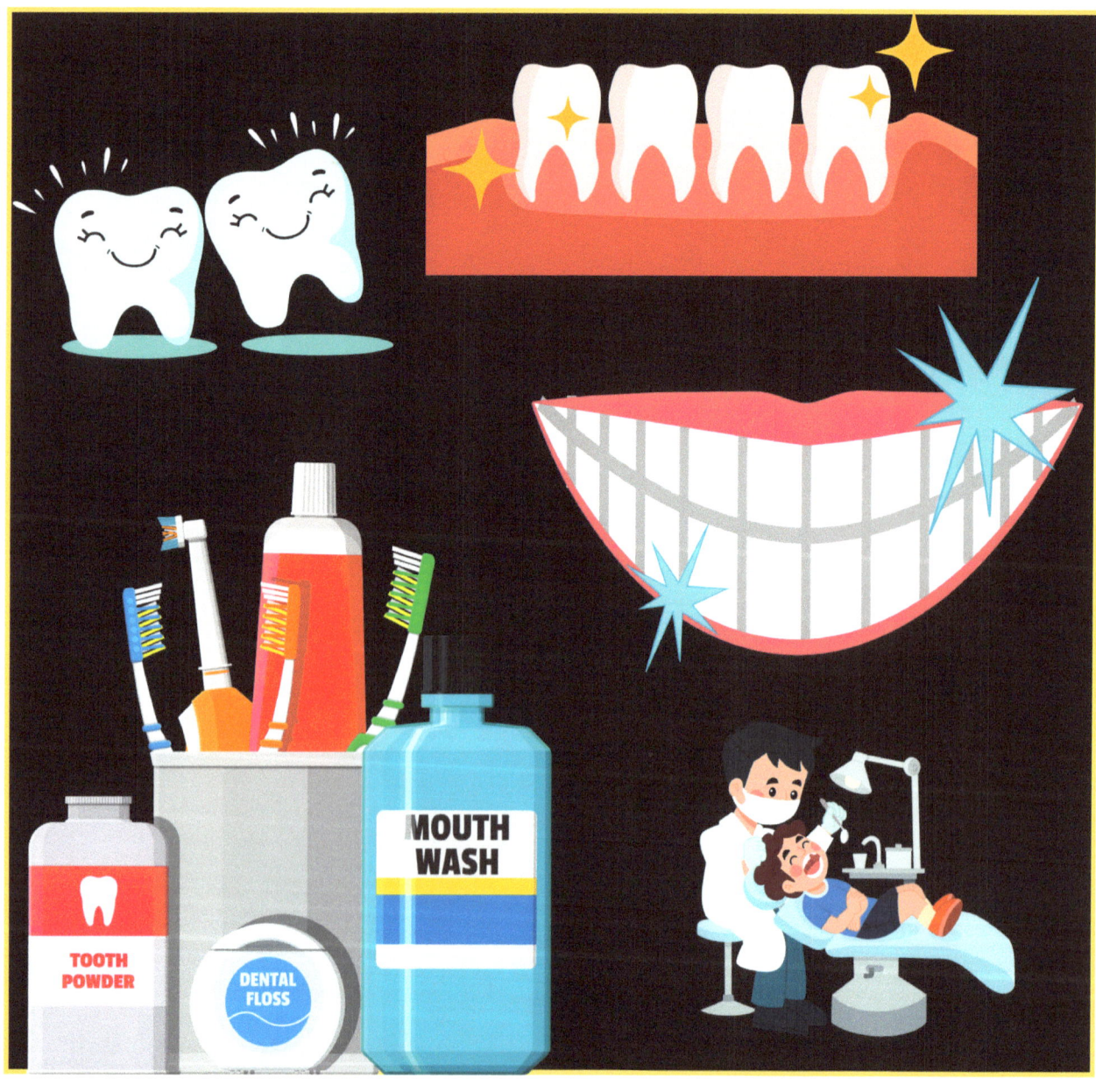

Z IS FOR ZYGOMATIC BONE

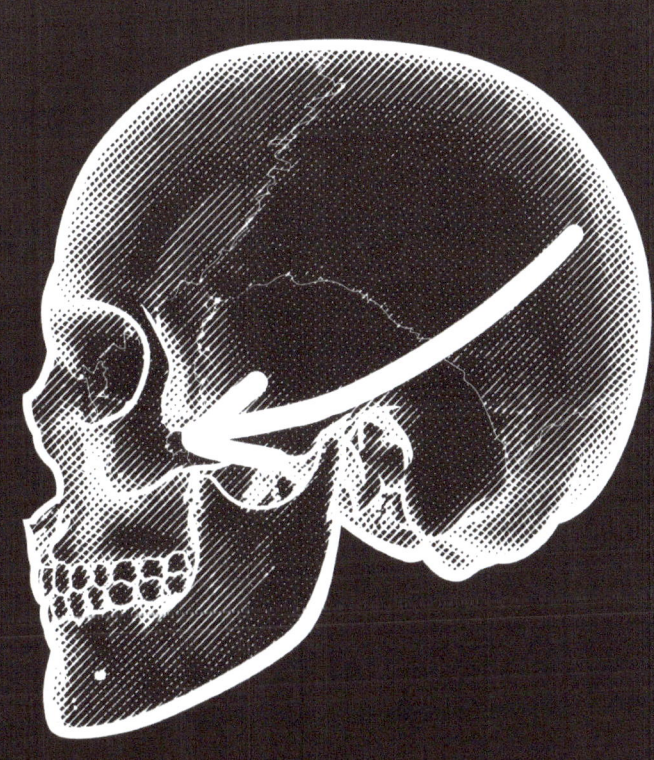

(Also known as cheekbone)

www.ingramcontent.com/pod-product-compliance
Lightning Source LLC
Chambersburg PA
CBHW060820290526
45792CB00005BB/1728